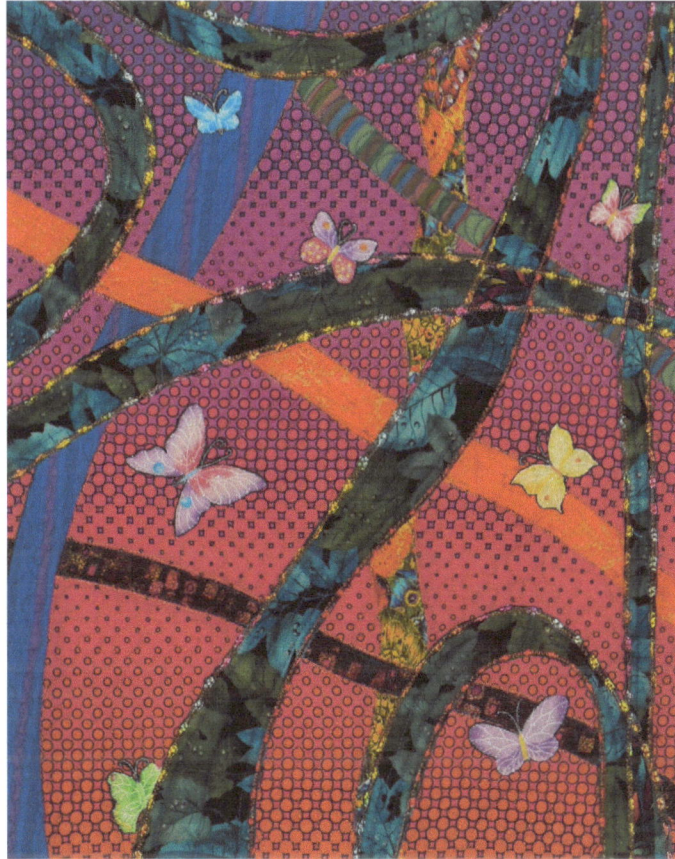

Healing Journey
by Lauren Kingsland
Quilts inspired by patients, caregivers and staff at
Lombardi Comprehensive Cancer Center at Georgetown University Hospital

Lauren Kingsland

Contact the artist/author at books@laurenkingsland.com
See more about her at www.laurenkingsland.com

CQS Press
Gaithersburg, MD

ISBN:0978704452
ISBN-13:978-0978704452

About the collection

A quilt can be a metaphor for putting together the pieces of a situation in an harmonious way. As an artistic medium, a quilt can be a tool for gaining a new perspective on the familiar. Each fabric alone can suggest an idea or evoke a feeling. Put them together in a quilt and often the result is a whole greater than the sum of its parts. The underlying message of a quilt is about the creation of beauty in daily life, about being tucked in and cared for, and about connection, cooperation and community. Almost everyone has a quilt story, whether they own one, have slept under one, or watched one being made by a family member. These roots in intimate domesticity make the quilt an ideal lens through which to look at the experience of cancer, or any illness.

These quilts were first exhibited as a group in the Atrium Gallery at Lombardi Comprehensive Cancer Center at Medstar Georgetown University Hospital, Washington, D.C. in October 2013. The pieces in this "Healing Journey" exhibit were inspired by the experiences of cancer that I have witnessed between 1998 and 2013 during my work at Lombardi as one of the professional visiting artists for the Arts & Humanities program. Each week I offer hands-on quiltmaking and fiber art projects to patients, families/ caregivers and hospital staff as a creative outlet for stress management and community connection. The motto of the hospital is *curae personalis*, care of the whole person. While the medical staff cares for the body of the patient, the artists are part of the medicine for the spirit. The presence of artists in the clinic is a reminder that Life is still large, even in the presence of a serious medical situation. Literally hundreds of people have sat with me through the years and shared their stories over pieces of bright colored cloth and a needle. In preparing this exhibit I returned to my journals and notes about the experience of being that listener. The "both/and" themes of courage and fear, connection and isolation, hope and anxiety, tranquility and busyness, which all ultimately lead to transformation, have emerged and shaped themselves into these visual images. I invite you to come along on this journey.

Lauren Kingsland

Alligator Mandala
24" x 24"
Cotton fabric, wool yarn, metallic thread, glass button

The healing journey is not a vacation trip with a preplanned itinerary and booked reservations. It is going into the unknown regions of self discovery. A diagnosis means that the old way of walking through life must change and the new way is not clear. Old maps of exploration often were decorated with a "compass rose" motif in the corner that showed the four directions, North, South, East, West, as a tool to help travellers figure out where they are and point the way to wherever they are going.

Some of those old maps also included warnings, such as "there be monsters here". This piece is to acknowledge that every healing journey involves facing the fear of the unknown. It may remind the viewer that guidance, directions and assistance are available for making that journey. Acknowledging the apprehension in the face of the unknown is the beginning of courage. There are monsters and we have to go anyway.

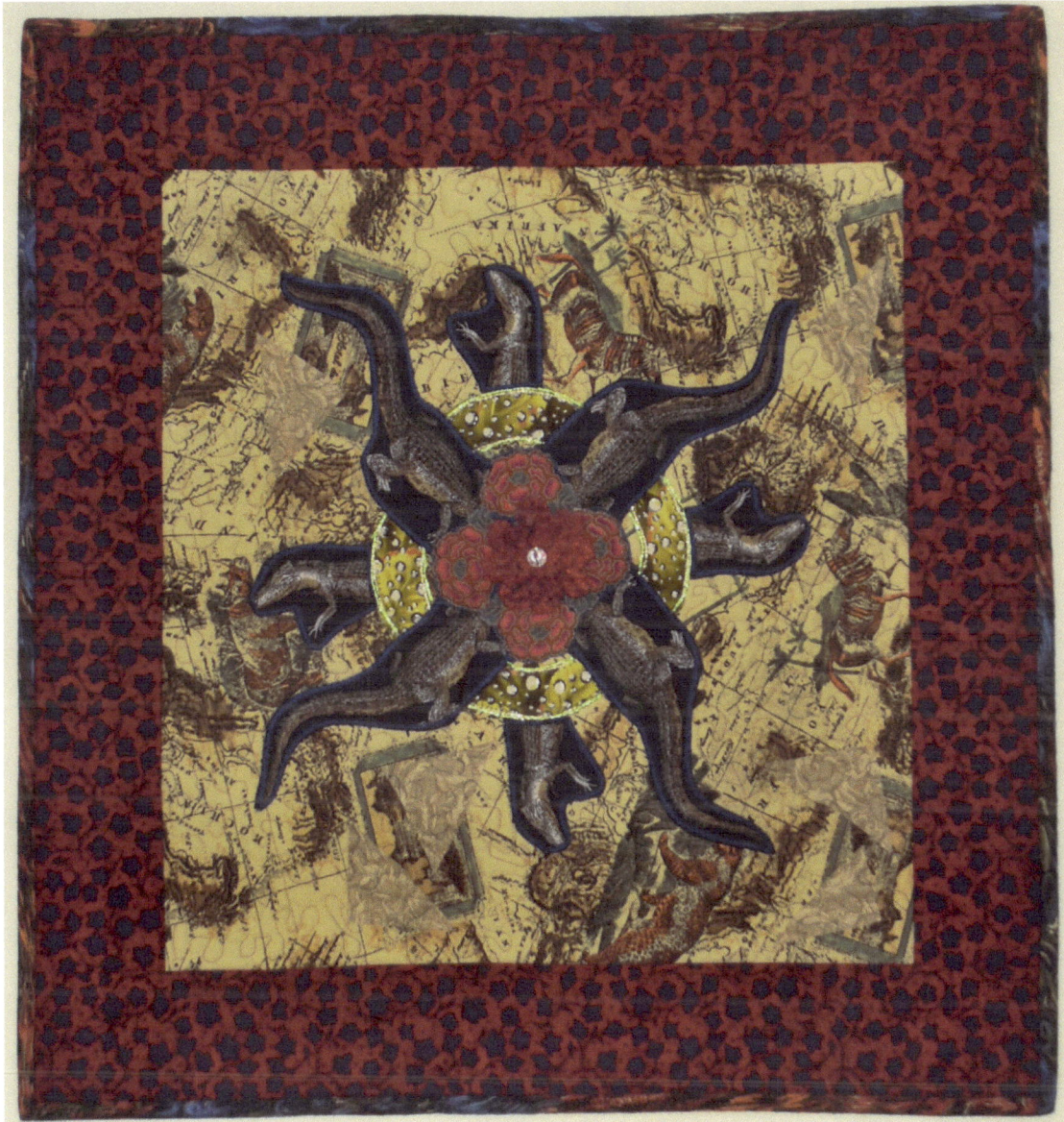

Aloft
19" x 17w"
Cotton fabric, rayon embellishment

These butterflies are flying above and through paths going every which way, oblivious to the confusion around them. Years ago I worked with the mother of a young man who was being treated for leukemia in a research unit at Lombardi. At that time there was a quiltmaking project for the staff and patients of that unit to make small quilts to brighten up those treatment rooms. This mother used her time waiting with her son by piecing and beading butterfly quilt blocks for the project, one after another. She said they represented her hopes for her son's return to health. They were part of her own healing process. Today her embellished butterflies adorn a folding screen in the corner of the Lombardi Clinic waiting room, for the benefit of other patients who also sit and wait and hope.

The butterfly is a symbol of transformation and continuity in the cycle of life. The egg hatches, the caterpillar eats and grows and gathers strength, the cocoon rests, the butterfly soars, and pauses to lay the eggs that allow the cycle to be repeated. For many people the butterfly is a symbol of the spirit; beautiful, resilient and flying free.

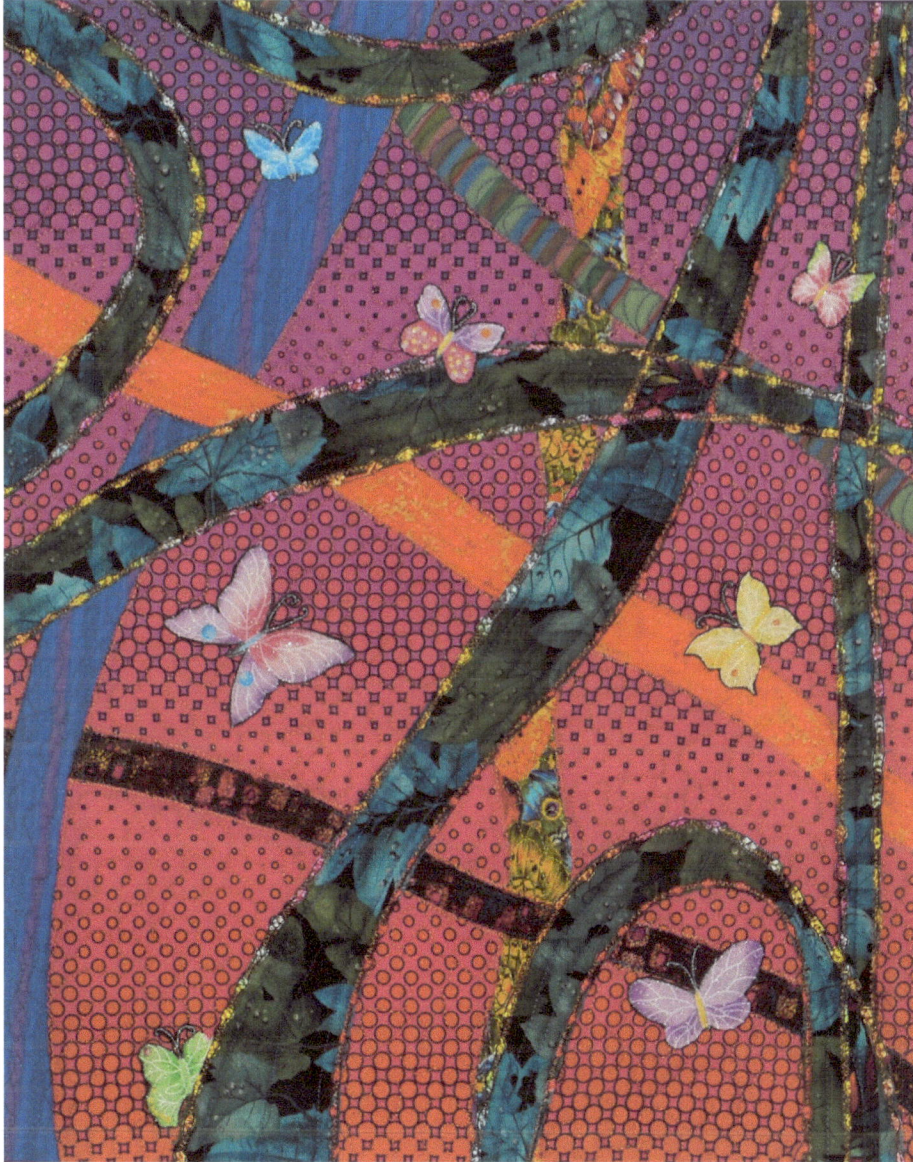

Cycles and Cycles
29" x 26"w
Cotton fabric, tulle, sequins and beads

The spiral is symbolic of movement. It is the simplest form of the contemplative labyrinth in which a walk in and back out on the circular pathway can produce an inner journey. When we move our bodies, our minds also shift. And we do not need to walk a path to experience this effect. Even tracing a spiral with a finger can be enough focus our attention. By going into "the heart of the matter", whether physically or in our minds, we can come back out with a new understanding.

Circles and spirals also remind me of the cycles of the seasons and of "both/and" thinking. Duality is always present: light and dark, rising and falling, growth and decay. This piece is based on a color progression used to describe the Chinese Five Element philosophy of cycles and interconnections which underlies the practice of acupuncture. This cycle model may be applied to describe the flow of the energy pathways in the body, or the course of a day, a relationship, a project, or an illness and return to health. This was part of my training in Applied Healing Arts at the Tai Sophia Institute/Maryland University of Integrative Health. My own work is with a different kind of needle and is yet another way to set up the conditions for change.

The colors here flow from one to another around the circle. Each represents a season, an element, an emotion, a phase. Blue is Winter, the water element, a time of dormancy and not knowing. Green is Spring, the element of wood, a messy time of beginning, new growth. Red is Summer, the fire element, a time of passion, rapid development, blooming. Yellow is Late Summer/Harvest, the earth element, the time of completion, ripening, acknowledgment and gratitude. White is Autumn, the metal element, the time of letting go, of grief, and of scattering the seeds that will come up again in Spring after the dormancy of Winter.

In the presence of cancer, it is helpful to recall that we are always somewhere in the larger cycle in our healing journey. We will not always be where we are today.

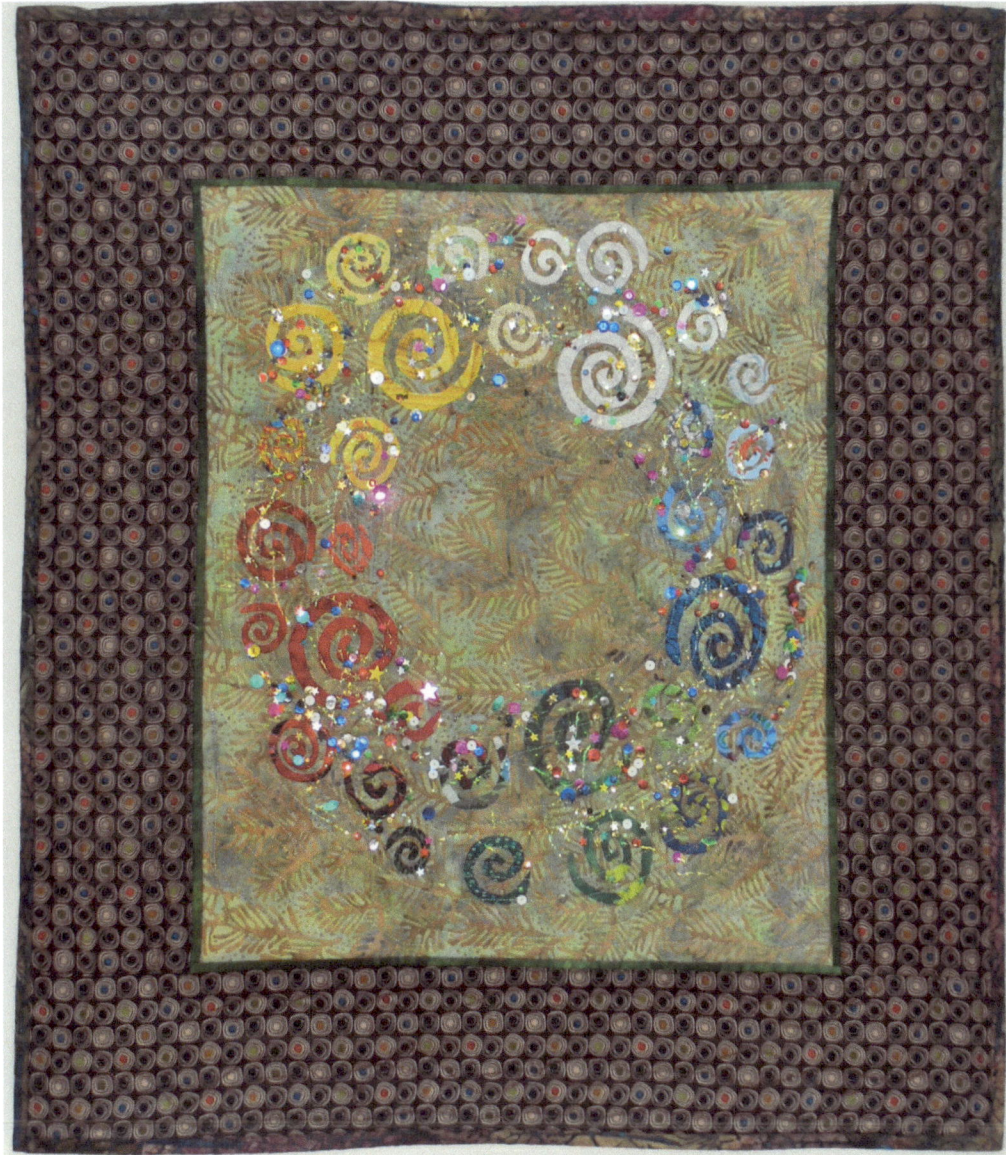

Treatment
29" x 29"
Cotton fabric, metallic thread, ceramic beads

The miracle of healing can happen as our bodies respond to various forms of medical intervention. Today's treatments offered to combat cancer come from years of dedicated, persistent, and creative research and experimentation by hundreds of people. Surgeries, infusions, radiation and medications are a real part of the landscape of the journey through cancer. The various design elements on this 9 point kaleidoscope design allude to these treatments, with sharp red-edged shapes, tubes weaving in and out, circular pills, and suggestions of structure and progression. This is to acknowledge and honor the medical community for generations of dedication to healing, and the courage of patients in undergoing treatment.

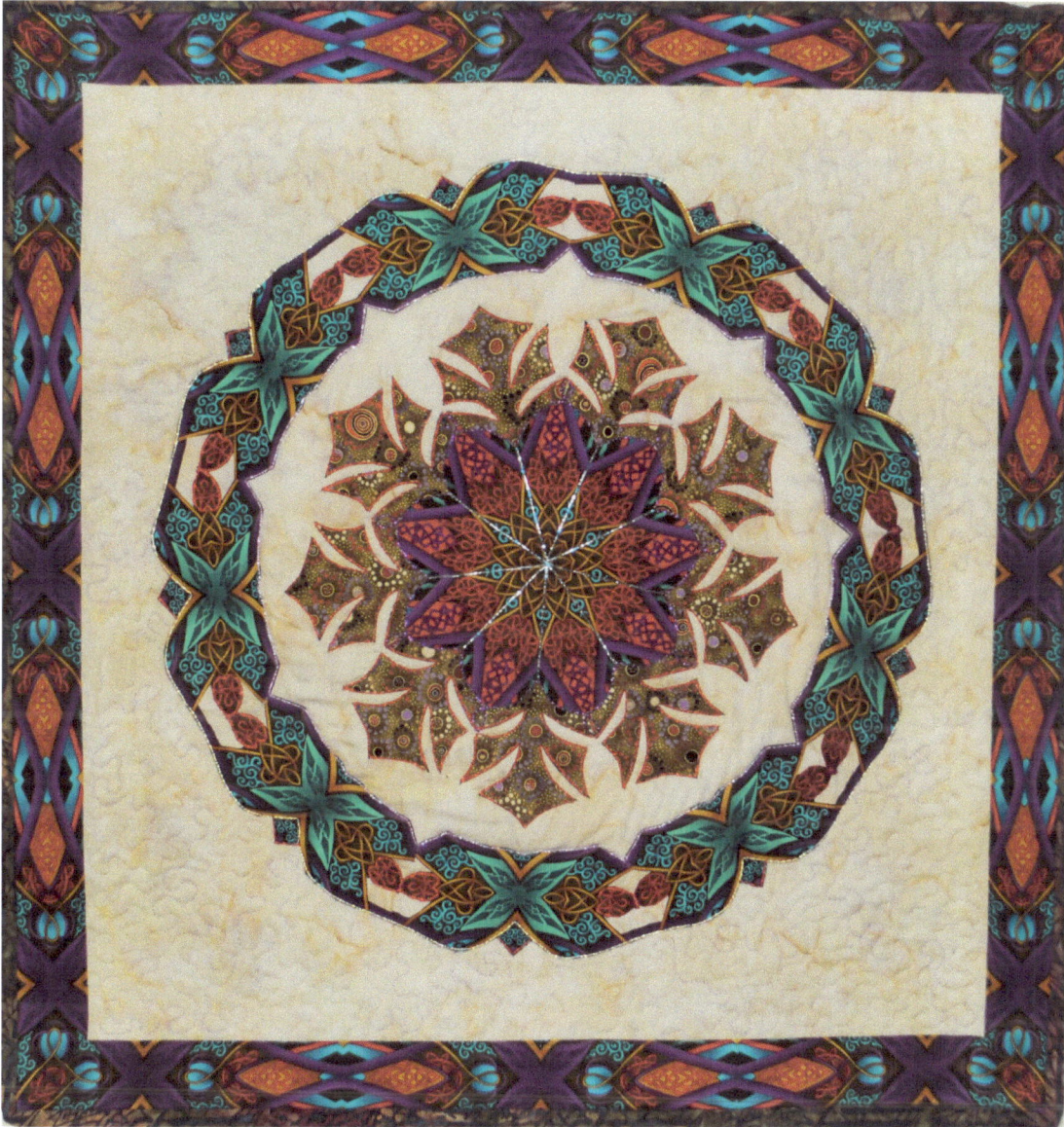

Heart's Journey
25" x 23"w
Cotton fabric, metallic thread, glass button

No one walks alone through the experience of cancer. It is a group pilgrimage including not only the patient but spouses, family members, friends, caregivers, medical staff and the wider community. Patients often tell me about how much they appreciate the people who come with them to clinic, call, visit, and stay in touch while they are being treated. Over and over I have heard, "Now I know what is really important in life - my family and friends." The heart shaped spiral represents a secure loving pathway over and against the background that contains little crabs within the flow of life, going about their business oblivious to anything else.

Why crabs? The ancient Greek physician Hippocrates, in 400 BCE, was the first writer to use the term *KARKINOS*, the crab, to describe what we today call cancer. Tumors with visible blood vessels reminded him of the many legged creatures in the sand, hence our term "carcinoma". Humankind has dealt with cancer for a long time.

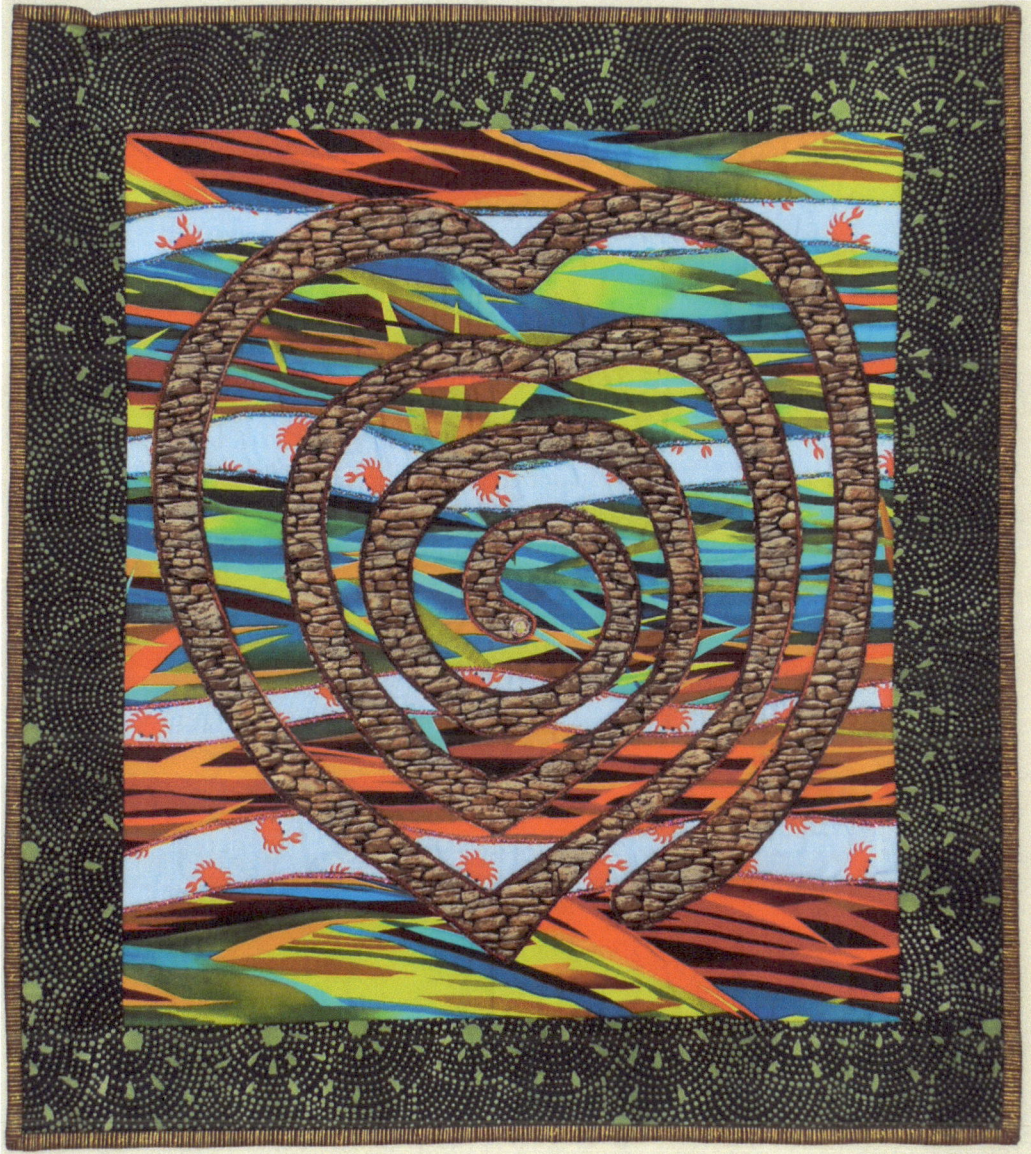

Constellations
27"x 24"w
Cotton fabric, metallic thread

This quilt is a companion piece to Heart's Journey. The brown stone wall has an opening in it that is the inverse or opposite of the path of loving companionship over a difficult place in Heart's Journey. The wall can stand for the security, or the confinement, of the assumptions each of us holds about how we think life is supposed to go. A serious illness challenges our underlying personal beliefs and stories about living. In this quilt the breach in the wall illustrates an expansion of understanding, represented by the stars including the constellation "Cancer", glimpsed through the opening. Patients often speak of a new understanding of how to live as a result of their illness, of deepened faith and hope, and of deciding to change how they use their time. In the aftermath of cancer, patients and survivors often make a new life for themselves. I have heard stories of career changes, new efforts to give back and support others in need, revisiting of artistic passions, and world travels. The possibilities are endless.

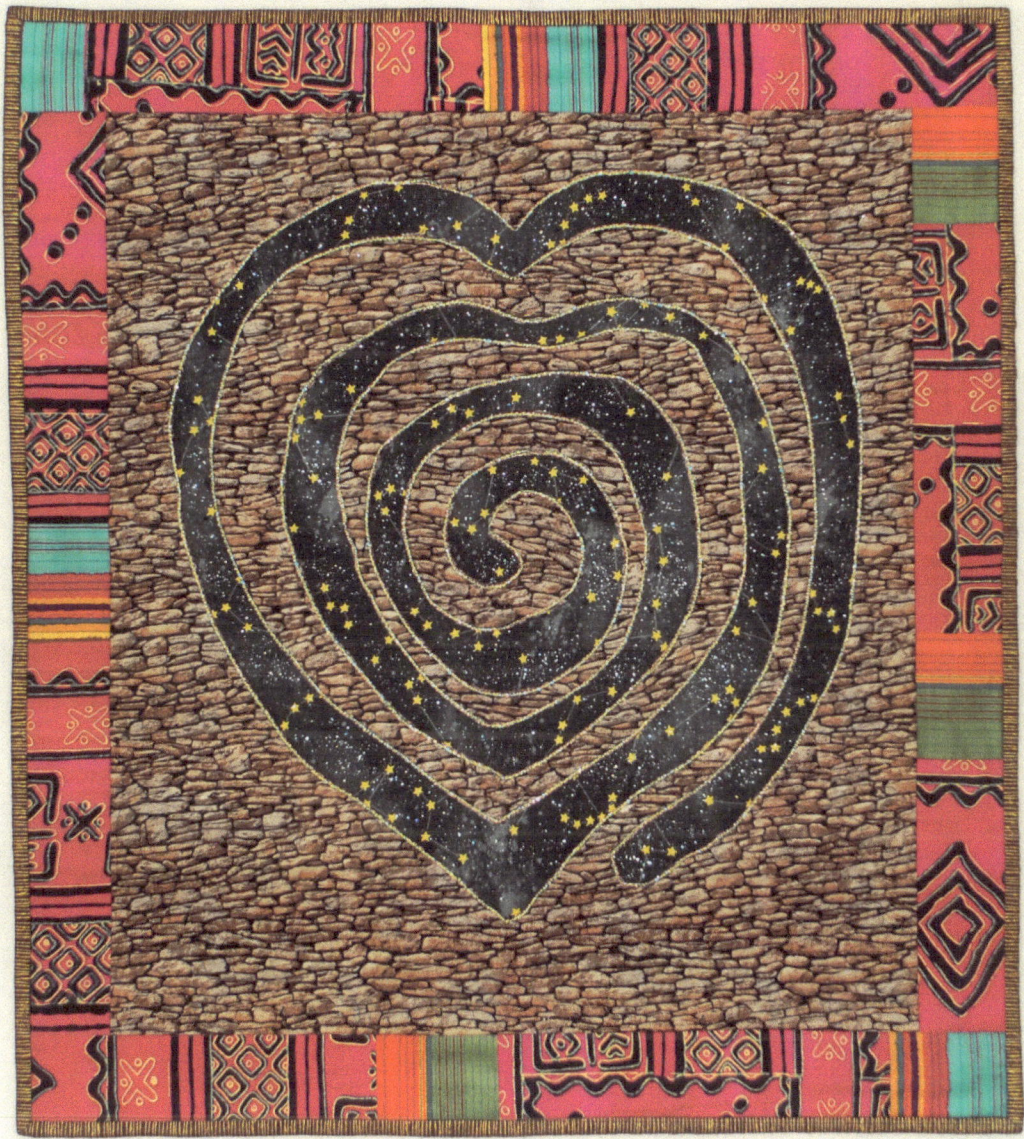

Beside Still Waters
29" x 26"w
Cotton fabric, metallic thread, jewel embellishments

The *kolam* is a traditional decorative practice of the women of Tamil Nadu, South India, drawn in rice flour on the ground at the doorway each morning as a painted prayer. I came upon this drawing tradition while traveling in India in 2008 and was enchanted. These designs show up in my artwork and in my daily journals as a tribute to our human delight with complexity, symmetry and closure. Balanced arrangements of continuous lines enclose every reference dot, with no loose ends, nothing left out, and no back-tracking. Using these simple rules there are dozens of variations possible for these apparently simple designs. In the same way, each day is like all others, and also unique and different from any other day that ever was.

Imagine this interlaced *kolam* design dropped gently onto the surface of a pool of still, pure water with dappled sunlight filtering through the leaves. Our bodies are mostly water. Even the idea of the presence of tranquil water can be very soothing. Peaceful water is a reminder of the mysterious ability of the body to use treatments to restore our health, balance and wholeness. The title is a reference to Psalm 23.

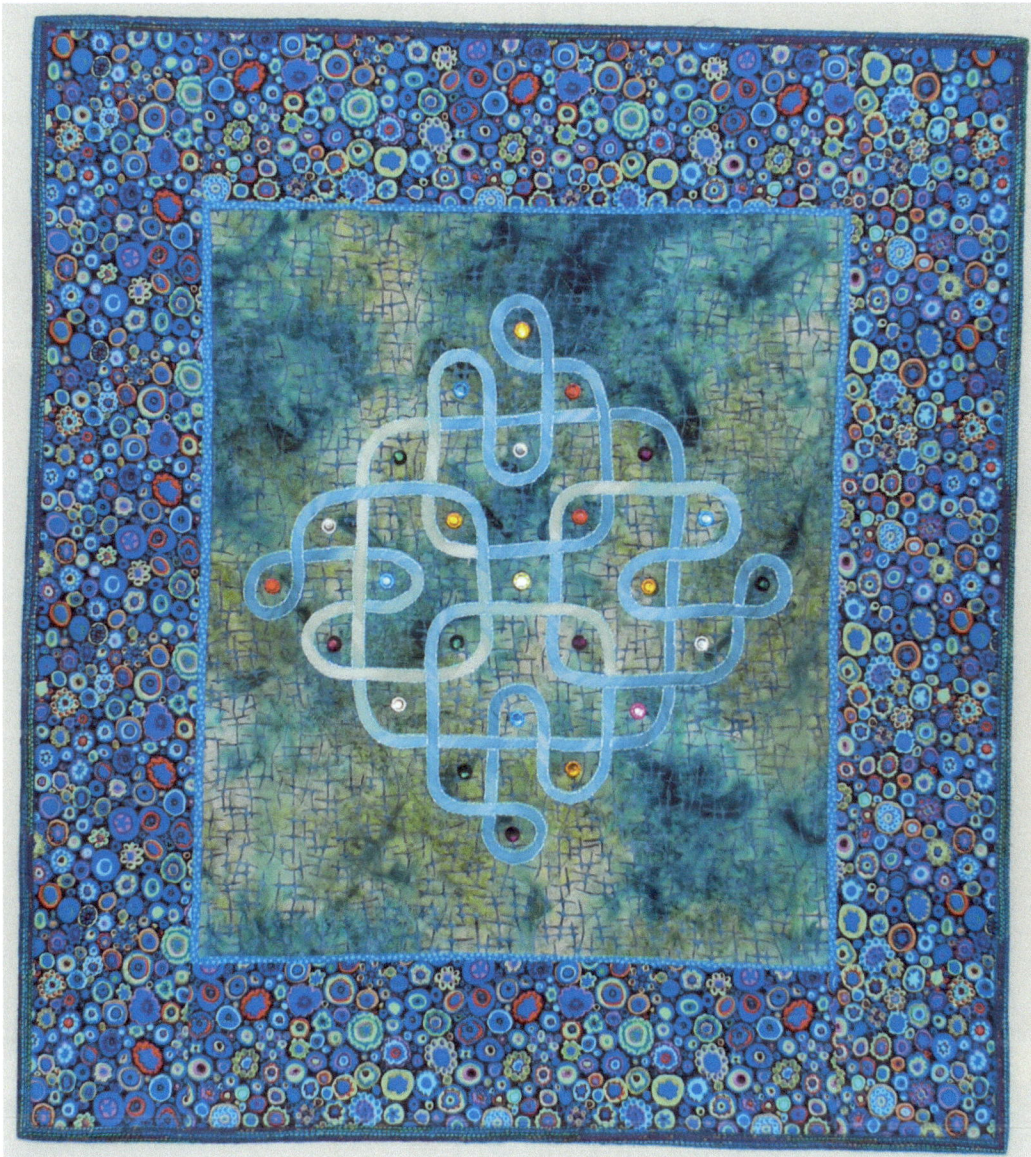

Lotus Panel with *kolam*
28" x 24"w
Cotton fabric, metallic thread, glass beads, mother-of-pearl button

Many treatments for cancer are derived from medicinal plants from around the world, symbolized here by this huge lotus flower. This central panel was hand drawn and hand dyed with natural dyes using a resist process by an artisan in India. I purchased it from him and added the borders, quilting and embellishments. The decoration in the corner is an example of another style of *kolam*. The design is one continuous line without visible reference points and is often referred to as the lotus. This is a reminder of our connection with the natural world and with other people around the planet.

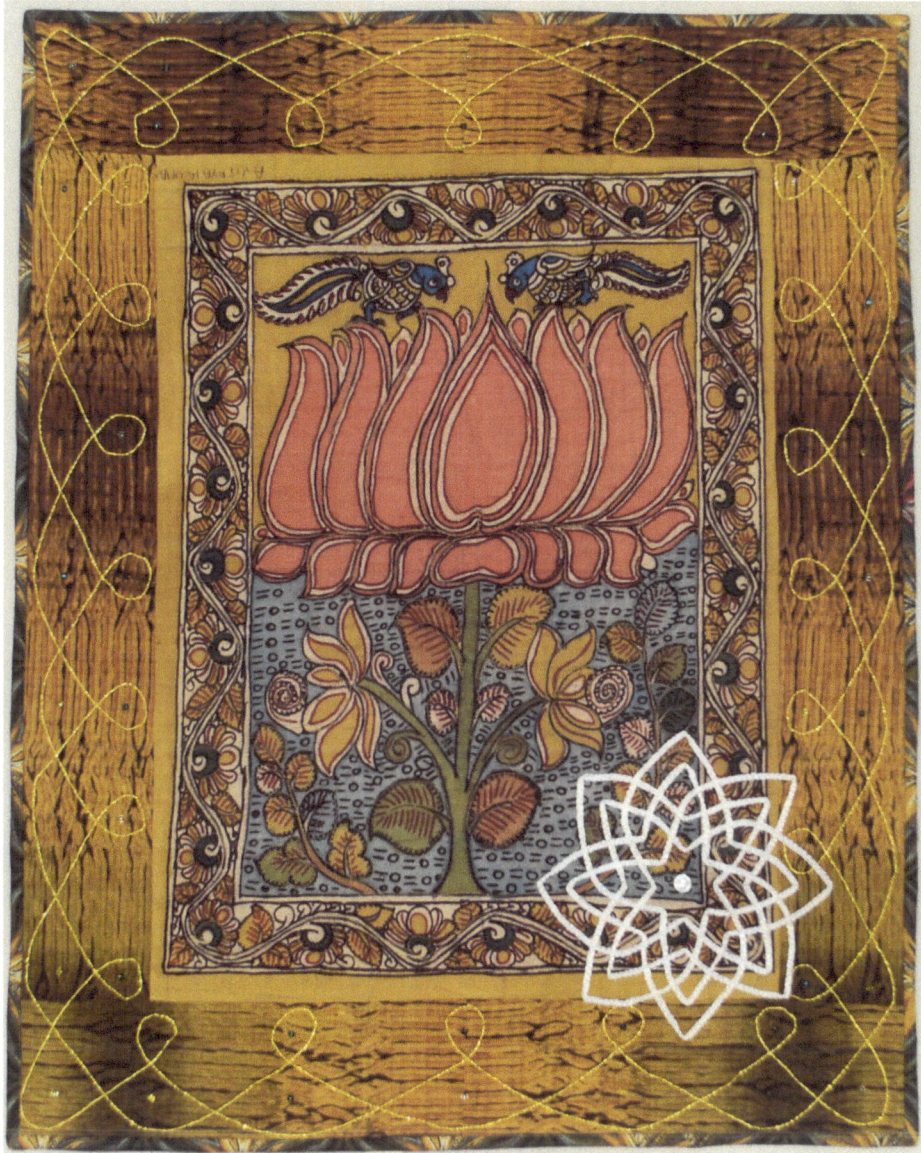

Tender Places
29" x 26"w
Cotton fabric, assorted buttons

This complex design is based on the South Indian *kolam* tradition of creating a daily drawing on the ground at the doorway as a contemplative practice. Reference dots are laid out in a grid to represent the concerns and gratitudes of that day offered up in prayer while preparing the drawing. The symmetrical continuous line around those dots is a reassurance that there is a way through what is present in that day which comes out right in the end, through many twists and turns along the way. The different buttons here are the many things to be faced by the viewer. This particular collection of buttons arrived as an anonymous gift left on the worktable in my public studio.

While going through the journey which is cancer, it is helpful to acknowledge and name the fears, concerns and reasons for thankfulness every day, and to hold to the knowledge that there will be a way through all of them. Remember that there are many right ways to go around what is present. Even if drawing a complex line is not part of the routine, writing in a daily journal about what is true now, and how one intends to deal with those things today is a valuable exercise for patients, families and caregivers.

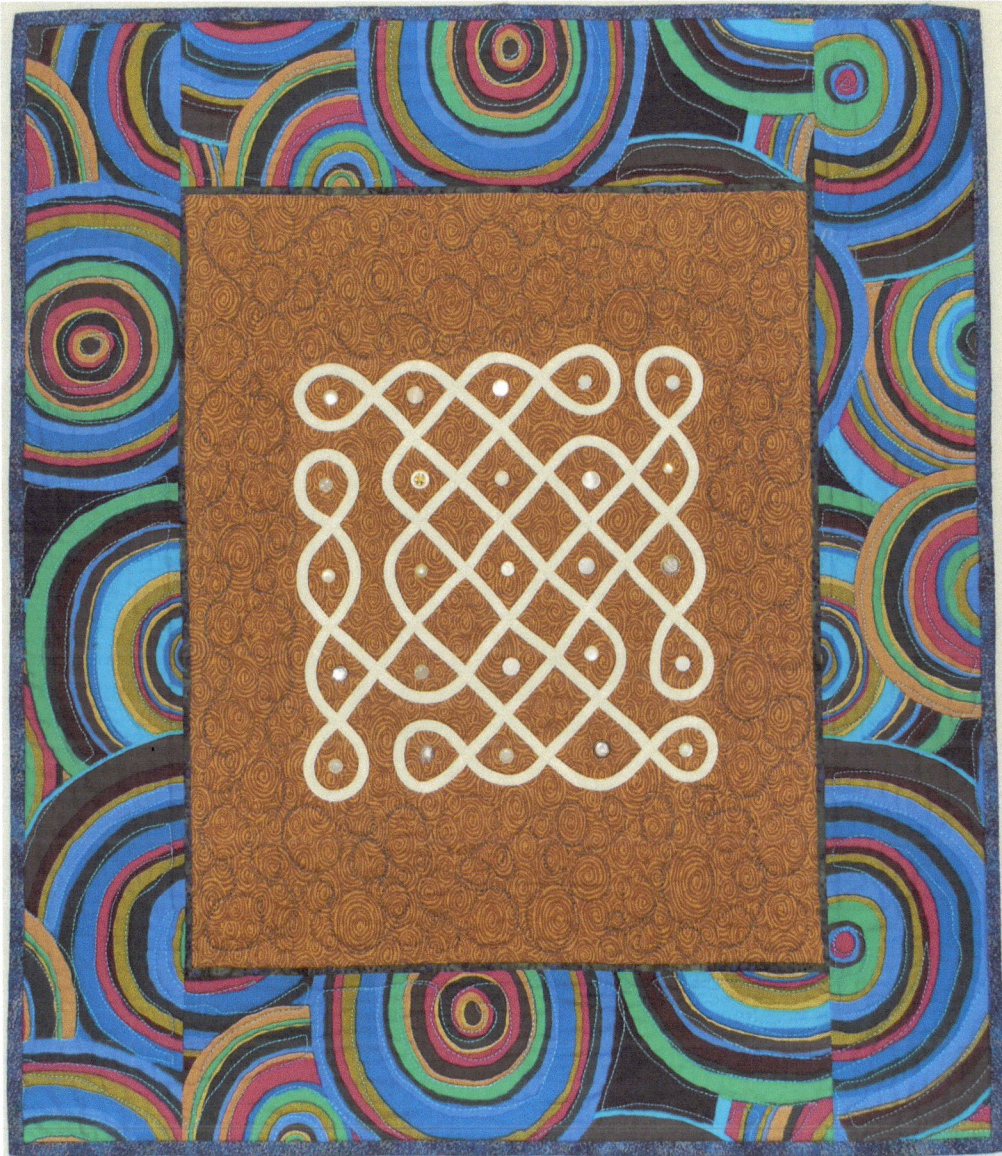

Fan Dance
29" x 26"w
Cotton fabric, plastic buttons

This quilt contains a personal story of my own journey that began in childhood. My parents were not connected in any way with the medical profession. My Dad was an engineer and my Mom was a piano teacher and editor. On the side however, my parents had a vision that convalescence in the hospital could be a time for creative handwork to occupy the mind and the hands. They developed a line of beaded flower kits to be sold in hospital gift shops. Those kits included buttons that looked like the center of a flower. The business remained very small and eventually they turned their attention to other pursuits. A small carton of glass beads, buttons and a few kits from "The Greenhouse Kit Company" has travelled through time with me. Some of those same buttons are the reference points in this *kolam*. I usually use white mother-of-pearl buttons on these pieces in this series but the dark background seemed to call for something else. I remembered the box of kit parts and dug out the yellow flower-center buttons. It was not until I rediscovered that box and put these buttons on this piece that it dawned on me that my work in arts in healthcare is the fruit of that dream my parents had of creative work as a component of healing.

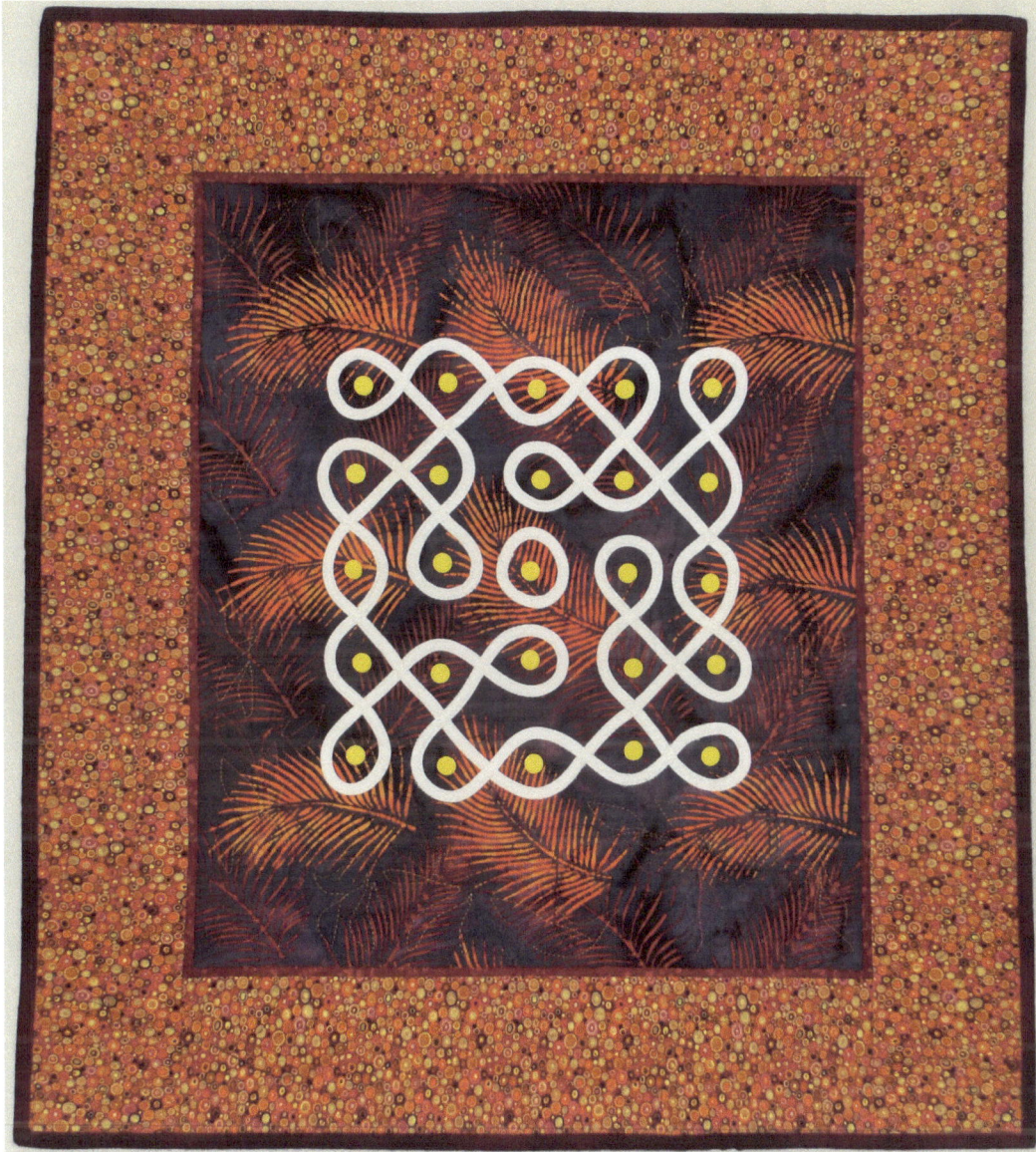

Fruits of the Spirit
44" x 44"
Thai silk, cotton fabric, rayon tape, glass beads

Laid onto a background of handmade Thai silk, this *kolam* design symbolizes the patterns of our life journey from day to day, each beautiful and complex, moving gracefully from one to the next. As my teacher Dianne Connelly used to say, "This is not a one-walk dog", meaning we may have to do the same thing over and over, day after day, to deal with the challenges we face. To create this complex pattern on the fragile silk required patience, mindful attention and persistence which are also qualities necessary also for the journey of healing.

The Bible, in Galatians, refers to the fruits of the Spirit as "Love, joy, peace, long-suffering, gentleness, goodness, faith, meekness, temperance...". In passages like this many people find strength and courage through the language of their religious faith to help them get through each day. The patients in the clinic who have shared with me through the years often speak, in their own way, of their deepened reliance on God as part of their experience with cancer.

The healing journey through these quilts begins with the compass rose image of the Alligator Mandala as a reminder that there is guidance. Fruits of the Spirit offers encouragement that although the road is long and difficult, there is much to be learned along the way. I have witnessed physical changes in individual patients over time as a result of disease and treatment. And I have observed that deep connection with others, inner growth, and transformation also happen during the experience of cancer. Each person walks in his or her own way through what they have to face to reach their own place of understanding, balance and hope. Safe travels.

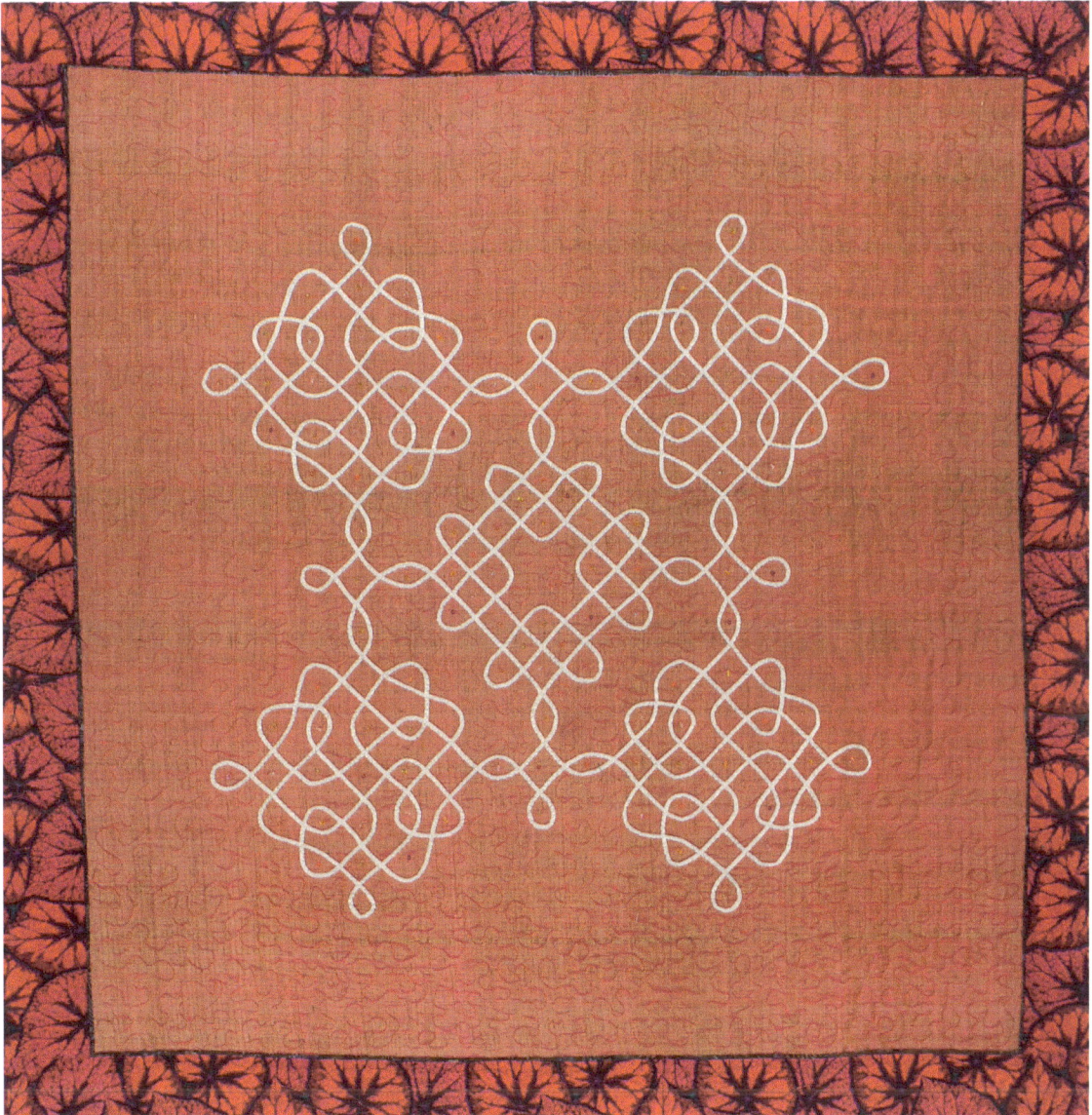

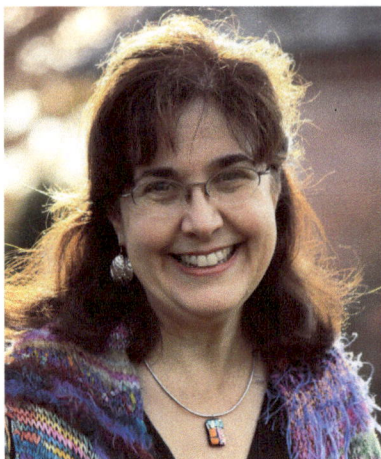

About the artist/author

Lauren Kingsland is a fiber artist, teacher, lecturer, author and artist-in-residence in the Sandy Spring Museum, Sandy Spring, MD. Her artwork is exhibited frequently in art spaces throughout the region. She provides hands-on workshops and lectures to medical, quilt and civic groups. Her arts in healthcare career began at the Clinical Center at NIH as a consultant to the Therapeutic Recreation staff at the time of the first AIDS quilt projects. She supports the Childrens' Inn at NIH as an founding art committee member and fundraiser. As the first professional Visiting Artist for the Arts & Humanities program at Lombardi Comprehensive Cancer Center at GeorgetownUniversity Hospital, she continues to offer fiber art projects as a creative outlet to patients, staff and caregivers. She holds a BA from Stephens College, Columbia, Missouri and an MA in Applied Healing Arts from Maryland University of Integrative Health. She is the author of "The Extraordinary T-shirt Quilt - A Scrapbook You Can Sleep Under" and editor of "Sacred Threads Exhibition 2013". Her book, "Design Your Day", offers ways to use the *kolam* as a tool for mindfulness.

Acknowledgements

Thanks to Nancy Morgan, director of the Arts and Humanities program at Lombardi Comprehensive Cancer Center at Medstar Georgetown University Hospital, Washington, D.C. for her ongoing support. This exhibit was created in response to her request for my work be exhibited during October 2103.

For the lessons in coming to life more fully to serve life more wisely, a deep bow to John Sullivan, Dianne Connelly, and to all the faculty and students in the Applied Healing Arts masters degree program at the Tai Sophia Institute, now the Maryland University of Integrative Health. Special thanks to John C. Wilson for his design help.

A shout out to the 20 plus other professional artists in the Arts and Humanities program at Lombardi. We are comrades in our worthy work to be the presence of the creative side of the human spirit in a challenging place where it is much needed.

My gratitude for the ongoing support and encouragement of Ben and Megan and Ivy Allen-Kingsland, Richard Bishop, Dr. Julie Bondanza, Carla Bonifasi, Patricia Dubroof, Kate Foley, Chappell Kingsland, Rosalind May, and Treva Miller.

Thanks to my parents, Ruth Lindal Swain and Pervis Alden Swain for their loving example of how to live abundantly and for starting me on this journey.

Photography by Megan Allen-Kingsland.